Stress

Two-minute Exercises to Break Up the Day

A Deskbook guide

NORMAL STRESS — OVER STRESSED — AFTER STRESS REDUCING EXERCISES

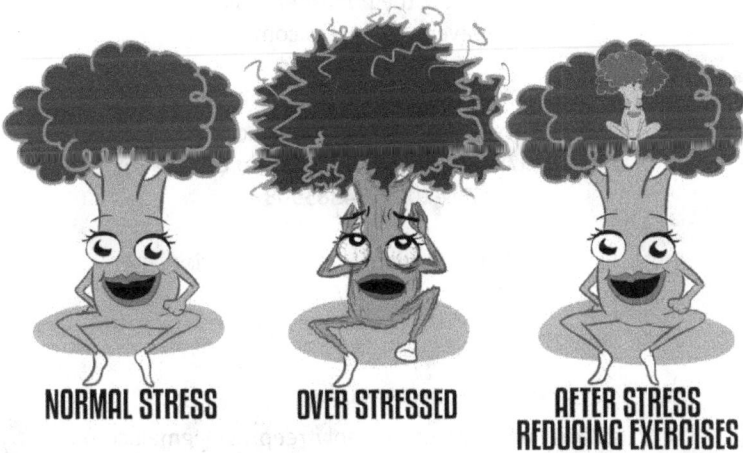

Cheryl Meyer – Cheryl M Health Muse
John Gins – Chun Mok

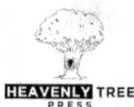

HEAVENLY TREE PRESS

For information, contact heavenlytreepress@gmail.com

DISCLAIMER

The content of this book is for general informational purposes only. It is not meant to be used, nor should it be used to diagnose or treat any medical condition or to replace the services of your physician or other healthcare providers. The advice and strategies contained in the book may not be suitable for all readers. Please consult your healthcare provider for any questions that you may have about your own medical situation. Neither the author, publisher, bodynbrain.com nor any of their employees or representatives guarantee the accuracy of the information in this book or its usefulness to a particular reader, nor are they responsible for any damage or negative consequence that may result from any treatment, action taken, or inaction by any person reading or following the information in this book.

DEDICATION

This book is dedicated to Scott and Junie Lee. They were the masters at our BodyNBrain Yoga Salon in Monrovia, CA.

Scott and Junie got us started on a series of stress releasing exercises in our weekly classes. I was to the point of extremely low cortisol from all the stress in my business, which was one reason I got autoimmune disease.

John suffered from a "frozen" shoulder.

By doing these exercises on a consistent basis, I was finally able to raise my cortisol level and release my stress before it became chronic. I learned to do these exercises intermittently on a daily basis.

John regained his flexibility in his shoulder and upper back.

Our masters were tapped by the worldwide Dao organization that BodynBrain was a part of, to open up the Eco Center in New Zealand for Ilchi Lee's organization. John continues to exercise virtually with their online class out of the Mago Center in Sedona, AZ.

I have added exercises that I learned in Airplane Aerobics on Northwest Airlines from my days of flying overseas to Asia. I added the Dr. Andrew Weil 4-7-8 - breathing exercise to my daily routine.

Learning these exercises has allowed my "leaky gut" to heal so that I no longer have pain from the autoimmune disease.

Both John and I are very grateful to Junie and Scott for their patience to get us back on track to return to wellness.

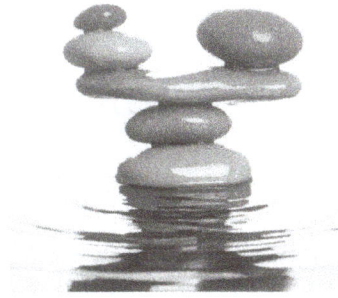

The World needs you at your Best

You are at your best when you resonate with your soul and focus in on your heart.

You are at your best when you are in balance and fully present in your life.

You are most productive when you release your stress throughout the day before it becomes chronic.

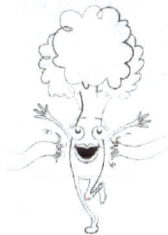

Let's discuss the importance of releasing stress for your health first:

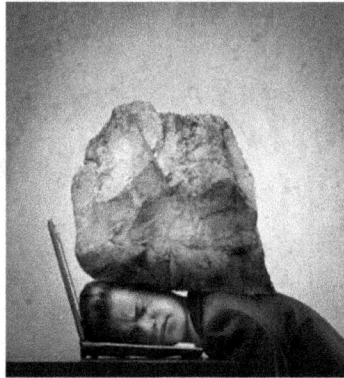

Chronic stress can affect every physical and psychological system. Its important to release your stress every day.

Chronic stress impacts the following:

- Heart Disease
- High Blood Pressure
- It breaks down the immune system and makes us susceptible to infection
- Stress contributes to "leaky gut," which leads to inflammation and pain. Stress releases inflammatory substances that travel through your body and attack body tissues. Stress causes disease.
- Stress causes muscles to tighten, and contract and over time creates back and neck pain and headaches

- Stress increases the permeability of the blood-brain barrier, allowing toxins, viruses, and poisons to flow through.
- Stress causes increased sugar cravings. Sugar is a toxin, as addictive as cocaine and which feeds cancer and causes inflammation. It turns off Ghrelin, a hormone that regulates appetite.
- Stress messes with your memory and brain functions.
- Stress causes weight gain and increased belly fat.
- Stress causes digestive issues.
- Stress reduces blood flow to the skin causing skin disorders (Psoriasis, Eczema, acne)
- Stress impacts mood, causing anxiety and depression.
- Most chronic illnesses have stress as one of their core issues. Stress creates "leaky gut," which is the root cause of chronic illness, and it wreaks havoc on all our major organs.

I had to learn to get my stress under control, or I couldn't get well. Quoting from my first book.[1] "My cortisol levels were low. Since I wasn't at 'disease' level, Addison's disease, then there was nothing to do, according to my conventional MD.

"My Functional MD ran a test for my DHEA level, which was completely depleted (DHEA is what the body uses to create new cortisol), she added a DHEA spray to my daily routine, increased my selenium, also good for my thyroid, had me work on my stress with exercise and breathing. The result: My cortisol is now creeping back into a healthier range.

"I reached a point where my DHEA was normal, but my cortisol was still low. I now use Rhodolia to keep my cortisol at more 'normal' levels."

Finding ways to reframe stress in our lives is crucial for reversing inflammation and squelching the degeneration of our tissues and the diseases of aging. Powerful stuff.

Recovery is not negotiable; you can either make time to rest and rejuvenate now or make time to be sick and injured later.

The long-term activation of the stress-response system and the overexposure to cortisol and other stress hormones that follow can disrupt almost all your body's processes. This puts you at increased risk of many health problems, including:

- Anxiety
- Depression
- Digestive problems
- Headaches
- Heart disease
- Sleep problems
- Weight gain
- Memory and concentration impairment
- Leaky gut and autoimmune disease

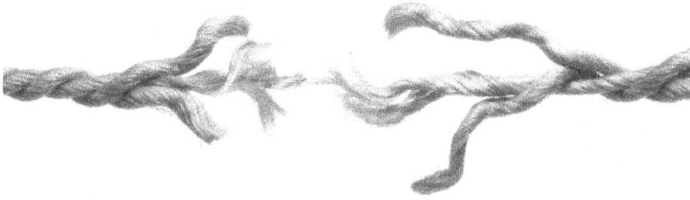

> "If you knew what was happening to your body when you're stressed out, you would freak out."
>
> Mark Hyman, MD

There is new ground-breaking research by Elizabeth Blackburn, Ph.D. the Nobel Prize winner who discovered telomerase and telomeres' role in the aging process and Elissa Epel, Ph.D., the health psychologist who has done original research into how specific lifestyle and psychological habits can protect telomeres, slowing disease and improving life. They concluded that "A telomere is a region of repetitive DNA at the end of a chromosome, which protects the end of the chromosome from deterioration." They continue, "Your telomeres don't sweat the small stuff.[2]

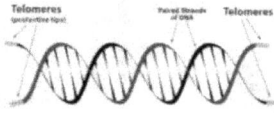

A Telomere is a region of repetitive DNA at the end of a chromosome, which protects the end of the chromosome from deterioration."

Telomeres don't sweat the small stuff

"Toxic stress, on the other hand, is something to watch for. Toxic stress is severe stress that lasts for years. Toxic stress can dampen down telomerase and shorten telomeres. Short telomeres create a sluggish immune function and make you vulnerable even to catching the common cold. Short telomeres promote inflammation (particularly in the CD8 T-cells), and the slow rise of inflammation leads to degeneration of our tissues and diseases of aging. We cannot rid ourselves of stress but approaching stressful events with a challenge mentality can help promote protective stress resilience in body and mind."

Finding ways to reframe stress in our lives is crucial to reversing inflammation and to squelching the degeneration of our tissues and the diseases of aging. Powerful stuff.

We accept that stress is very hard on the body and negatively impacts our health. The question becomes, how do we reframe our response to lower our stress level and its damage to our health? Because recovery is not negotiable, you can either make time to rest and rejuvenate now or make time to be sick and injured later. Imagine your health to be a cup of warm, soothing tea. Keep your cup full.

Chronic stress puts your health at risk

Your body is wired to react to stress to protect you from getting eaten by a tiger. Protection from predators is rarer in today's life, but the mechanisms are still in place and can be triggered by a variety of experiences.

Stress can accumulate from all areas of life, but one of the most common places to feel and increase our body's stress is in the workplace. The long-term activation of the stress-response system and the overexposure to cortisol and other stress hormones that follow can disrupt almost all your body's processes. This puts you at increased risk of many health problems, including:

- Anxiety
- Depression
- Digestive problems
- Headaches
- Heart disease
- Sleep problems
- Weight gain
- Memory and concentration impairment

Stress continues to accumulate in the body and must be released before it becomes "Chronic or Toxic."

Chronic stress leads to leaky gut

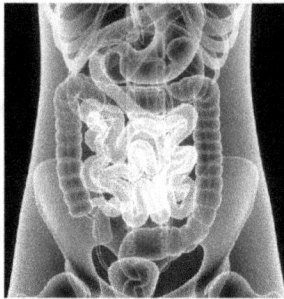

The bacteria in the gut break our food down into amino acids. A healthy gut lining allows friendly amino acids to go into our system as particles that are recognized by our immune system as friendly particles.

If our digestion isn't working properly, if we don't have enough "good" gut bacteria, large chunks of food are in the gut, not yet broken down into amino acids.

Leaky gut is where the link in the chain of your gut breaks, and tiny little holes allow these larger food particles to pass through the wall and into your bloodstream. These holes remain open, allowing the larger food particles to pass through. These holes need to be healed and closed for the disease to stop progressing.

Over time, you can build up antibodies against any food that is slipping through, chicken, tomatoes or a long list of other foods that are your sensitivities, so your immune system perceives more and more particles as the enemy.

Chronic stress is a contributing factor to Chronic Disease

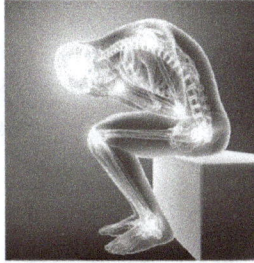

These particles do a form of molecular mimicry. Our immune system sees them as foreign invaders similar to other cells in the body. These particles could look like thyroid tissue or other tissues in the body, and our immune system then attacks not only the "foreign" invader, (the larger food particle that is slipping through) but also the tissue that is being mimicked. Our immune system starts to attack our own body. The immune system is signaled to attack different body systems, wherever our greatest vulnerability is and where the tissues being mimicked are.

For me, it was my muscles, my liver, and my pancreas. For someone else, it might be their thyroid. It is what causes MS and Lupus, and it is what causes Rheumatoid Arthritis and diabetes. It causes brain fog, and eventually, it causes Alzheimer's. It is now thought to be what causes Parkinson's. It might even cause autism. It causes healthy body functions to break down.

Stress can build up in all areas of life

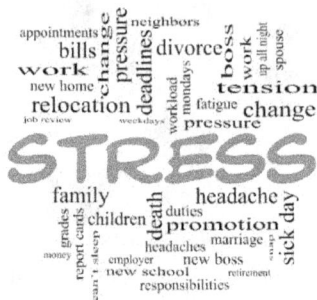

But the #1 area that we are under the pressure of stress is in the workplace. This is a desk guide to keep on your desk.

Exercises to improve body and mind balance

The major way we can control our stress is by quieting our busy brain and focusing on our bodies. In this section, we present methods that will help you raise your pulse, find your focus, and quiet your brain. One of the many benefits will be an increase in your productivity.

These exercises reduce stress, can be done anytime and anywhere. They should be incorporated into your daily lifestyle. They need no equipment.

BEFORE YOU RISE

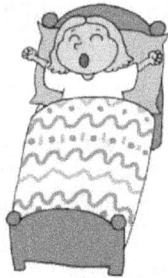

- Stretch from the tips of your fingers to the tips of your toes

- Take 3 deep breathes - Breathe in for a count of four and hold it for a count of 7 before you whoosh it out.
- Do a fast palm rub with your hands over your chest close to your body. Do this for 30 seconds. This will wake you up and send energy all over your body.

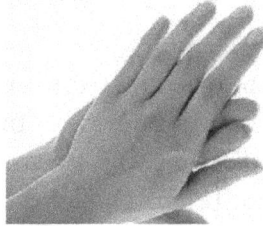

- Do the spinal twist. Bring your knees to your chest, and then take one leg across your other leg and twist your back while you extend the other leg out straight in front of you. Put your arms into a cactus position and turn your head in the opposite direction from the side your leg is on. Hold this twist for a count of 5. Breathe deeply. Breathe in for a count of four and hold it for a count of 7 before you whoosh it out. Switch and repeat on the other side.

WHEN YOU FIRST GET OUT OF BED

- Do 3 deep breathes.

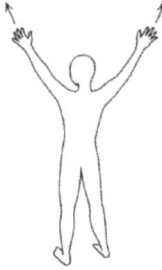

- Standing raise your arms above your head to touch the ceiling. Do 3 deep breathes.

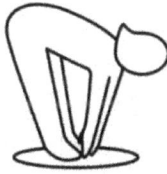

- Now bend down to touch your toes
- Do 3 deep breathes.

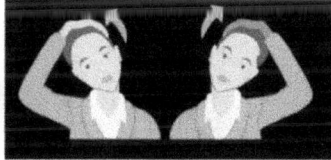

- Stretch your neck to the right and hold it for 5 seconds.
- Do 3 deep breathes.
- Stretch your neck to the left and hold it for 5 seconds.
- Do 3 breathes.

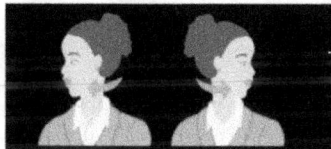

- Turn your head to the right, look over your shoulder and hold it for 5 seconds.
- Do 3 deep breathes.
- Turn your head to the left and look over your shoulder and hold it for 5 seconds.
- Do 3 deep breathes.

Now you are ready for step 2 of your morning routine

Step 2 Morning Routine:
MORNING

- Greet the Sunrise[3] - This could be as simple as looking out a window to view the Sunrise and expressing gratitude. Sunrise is my favorite part of the day, and its spectacularly different every morning.

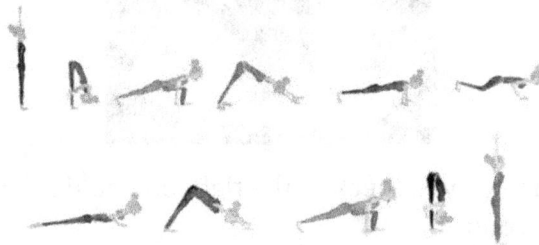

SALUTE THE SUN.

- You could also do the yoga routine to greet the sun.
- Morning papers[4]

"Morning Pages are three pages of longhand, stream of consciousness writing, done first thing in the morning. There is no wrong way to do Morning Pages - they are not high art. They are not even "writing." They are for your eyes only. Morning Pages provoke, clarify, comfort, cajole, prioritize, and synchronize the day at hand. Do not over-think Morning Pages: just put three pages of anything on the page. And then do three more pages tomorrow." These are "cloud-thoughts." "You are meeting your shadow and taking it out for a cup of coffee." It's a great way to clear out your "dark thoughts" before you start your day.

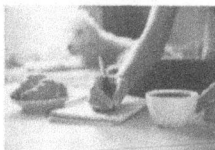

7 RULES FOR WRITING MORNING PAGES

1. WRITE EVERY MORNING

2. JUST WRITE

3. WRITE BLIND

4. IT IS WHAT IT IS

5. NO BACKTRACKING

6. KEEP IT PRIVATE

7. THERE ARE NO RULES

- List 5 things you are grateful for that morning

Record your Victories from the previous day and make a note of the 3 things you are grateful for that morning. You can record these in a notepad designated to this task, or you can purchase my journal designed for this purpose.

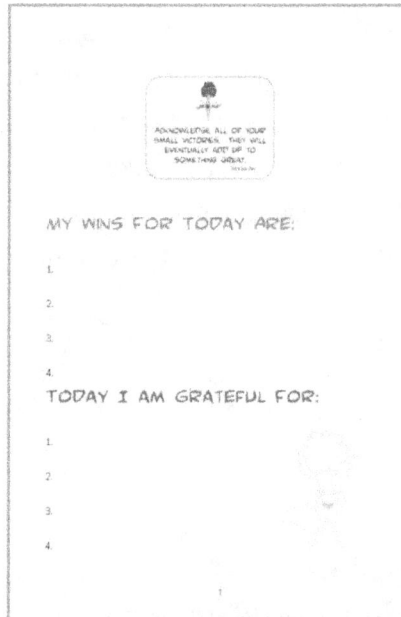

My book **It Feels Good to Feel Good, Daily Victory Journal** to Celebrate your Daily Wins and Practice Gratitude is a perfect place for your record all the things that are currently good in your life. Available on Amazon.

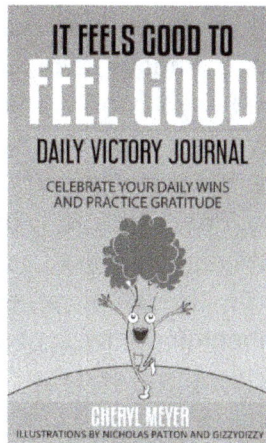

IT FEELS GOOD TO
FEEL GOOD
DAILY VICTORY JOURNAL

CELEBRATE YOUR DAILY WINS
AND PRACTICE GRATITUDE

CHERYL MEYER
ILLUSTRATIONS BY NICHOLAS PATTON AND GIZZYDIZZY

Stress builds up all day long. Every hour spend 1-2 minutes on releasing the build-up by using these methods. If you can't do one of every hour, at least do one 3 times a day. Set the alarm on your phone and choose times to do them. I do 11 AM, 2 PM, and 5 PM. The 2 PM is especially helpful right after lunch because it wakes my body and my brain up and increases my productivity.

ALL DAY - Choose One at a time to release your stress in 2 minutes.

Change these up and do them intermittently throughout the day.

- Dr. Weil's 4-7-8 breathing exercise 4 rounds at least 2x daily. This resets your parasympathetic nervous system. (Dr. Weil has a video on YouTube where you can do the breathing with him)
- Take your fingers and push into your belly button and just jiggle up and down for 1 minute. The theory is that your belly button is the beginning of

our life, and through our belly button, we can impact your entire body. If you are in a private space, use the Belly Button Wand (more details later.) But if you are in a public space, your fingers work just fine. This affects your reptilian brain at the back of your neck (the early brain in development) and significantly reduces your stress as proven by Dr. Emerel Mayer, executive director of the Oppenheimer Center for Stress and Resilience (uclacns.org) and the Co-director of the Digestive Diseases Research Center at the University of California at Los Angeles.

- Stand and bounce in place every hour to break up the day will bring energy to the brain. Stand up by your desk, let your arms hang, and bounce. Use your toes. Do this for 1-2 minutes
- Tapping the body starting at the ankles and working up to the top of the head. Don't hurry. Give each area of your body, loving attention.

Do front and back of your feet (don't forget the bottoms), your ankles (all the way around), your calves (the front and then the back), your thighs, (the front and then the back), your tummy (make a fist and pound your tummy with them firmly but not hard), your heart zone (tap all over your chest), now tap your shoulders, (Make sure you get the front and the back), go down one arm, front and back and then back up, including your hand and then do the other, your face (gently tap it all over, including your ears) and then the top of your head. (Take your fingers and strongly tap on your head all over.) Go back down and tap your back where you can reach it and your butt. This should take 2 minutes. Each area would get about 6-10 seconds, so do not rush. You should be able to feel the energy all over your body when you finish.

Some people prefer to start their tapping from head to ankle. Adopt a method that works best for you.

- Every hour on the 1/2 hour, stretch at your desk. Be sure to stretch up and stretch out. You can do it seated, or you can stand. Each stretch should be long and slow. Start by stretching up. Hold it for 10 seconds, then stretch down. If you are standing, touch your toes and hold that for 10 seconds. Put your arms straight out like an airplane and stretch for 10 seconds. Now touch your ear to your shoulder on the left and hold it for 10 seconds, and then touch your ear on the right to your right shoulder and hold it for 10 seconds. Face forward - turn your face and look to the left without your body changing position and then face forward again, now turn your face to the right and hold it for 10 seconds getting nice long stretches. With your arms out in front of you, but parallel to the ground, bend your wrists and stretch out all your fingers for 10 seconds. Now do the same thing with your feet. Put your legs out straight and bend your ankles and stretch out all your toes.

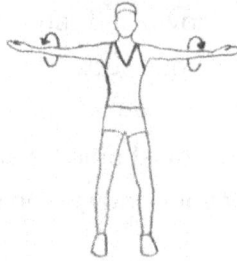

- Put your arms straight out. Roll your arms from the shoulder in large rolls. Do 10 forward. Reverse and do 10 back. Repeat 3 times.

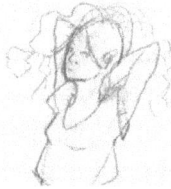

- Bend your arms and put your fingers next to your neck. Leading with your elbow, roll your arms forward 10 times and then roll your elbows backward 10 times. Do 3 sets. Release the tension in your upper back and shoulders.

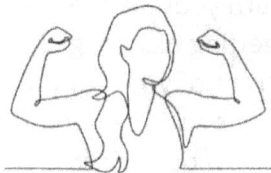

- From a seated position, put your arms straight out to the side in a straight line, and then bend them at the elbows like a goal post. Slowly bring your elbows together in front of your nose, and then open your elbows again. Do 10 repetitions.

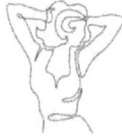

- Seated, put your hands behind your head and clasp your fingers. Your feet should be firmly on the floor. Twist to your right and hold the stretch for 5 seconds. Reverse and twist to the left and hold for 5 seconds. Repeat 3 times.

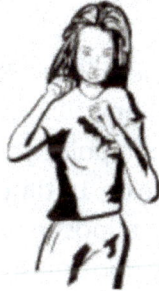

- Faux boxing- put your arms out in front of you while you are seated in your office chair. Make a fist with each hand. Bring your fists close to your body. Now alternating fists, hit an imaginary punching bag 20 times each side. Break-do 2 more sets.
- I just learned a new stress releaser that you do from a sitting position. Put your hands on the side of your thighs (at the same time, one hand on the outside of each thigh) push out with your legs as you push in with your hands. Hold for 10 seconds and release. Do it again. You will feel relaxation go through your entire body.
- Now do the opposite. Put your hands on the insides of your thighs. Push your thighs against your hands and build resistance. Hold for 10

seconds and then release. Do it again. Enjoy the tingling.

- When fatigued, toe-tap from a sitting position. Just put your legs out straight and tap your toes. Do this for 60 seconds. You may need to do this often to build up to a full minute, and if so, do this as long as you can.
- Open and close your hands 10 times, making a fist and then relaxing your hand, spreading out your fingers. Then roll your wrists 10 times in each direction.
- Now do the same things with your feet. Put your legs out straight and flex your foot up and widen the toes, and then point your feet flexing your toes. Now roll each ankle 10 times to the left and 10 times to the right, loosening up your ankle.
- Sitting in a chair, looking straight ahead, with your feet on the ground, raise your right heel up until you are bending your toes as far as you can. Push down on your toes. Count to 10. Lower your foot. Do the other foot. Do 10 reps of each 3 times. Stretching your toes this way relaxes your body. We hold a lot of our stress in our feet.
- Sitting in your chair, do seated hip marching. Put both feet flat on the ground, hold onto your seat, and lift your right knee as high as possible and hold for a count of 5. Now do the left side. Do 3 sets.
- Rest Your Eyes and Turn Off the Lights

I learned many of these exercises by doing yoga with Body and Brain Yoga. They have significantly lowered my stress. https://www.bodynbrain.com/ there is also an APP http://1minchange.changeyourenergy.com/

The Belly Button Wand is an excellent tool to release stress.[5]

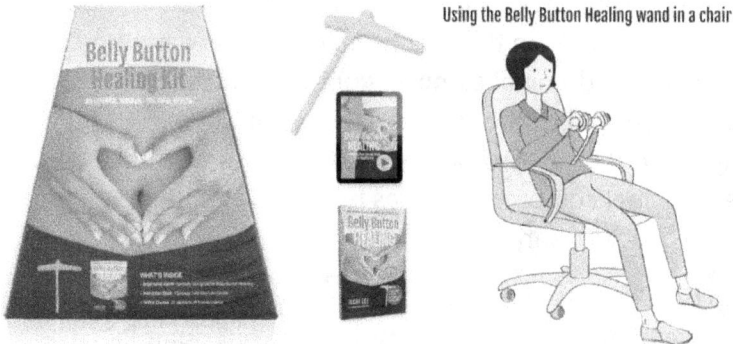

Using the Belly Button Healing wand in a chair

"Eastern medicine has known for thousands of years the importance of the belly button as an acupressure point. In fact, the belly button was even used as a stimulating point to revive someone in emergency treatment when a person suddenly lost consciousness or has collapsed due to high blood pressure or stroke!

"In Eastern medicine, the acupressure point in the belly button is known as "Shin-gwol," which means "the place where God resides." The belly button is the place where life starts and is received and transferred by the embryo via the umbilical cord in its mother's womb. Your belly button is not just a scar left over from birth! It is a very important acupressure point in recovering health and vitality."

The Belly Button Wand - Does it work?

Increasing Blood Circulation

A fascinating study reported by the Los Angeles Times and The Washington Post shows the effectiveness of stimulating the abdomen. Researchers from the St.

Joseph's Hospital and Medical Center in Paterson, NJ, provided treatment for resuscitating 103 emergency patients whose breathing was gradually stopping. There were two kinds of treatment: one was the conventional method of CPR on the chest; the other was a method that involved abdominal compressions in addition to traditional CPR. Amazingly, the recovery rate with the chest-CPR was no more than 7%, while the recovery rate with the abdominal compressions was more than triple that of only the chest at a surprising 25%.

So how does it work? Your gut holds one-third of your entire body's blood supply. When we put pumping pressure on the abdomen through Belly Button Healing, it circulates the blood collected around your vital organs throughout the entire body from head to toe. Regular blood circulation is the key to revitalized energy.

When you lack vitality or are feeling the afternoon slump, pressing on the belly button through Belly Button Healing can help your body recover vigor and warmth. The benefits of breaking up your day with mini stress releasing exercises.

By breaking up your day every hour with any of the above 1 to 2-minute mini exercises:

- You send blood to your brain, release the stress, and relax.
- You also wake your body up to feel alive.
- You will think better and be more productive.
- You will improve your digestion and reduce the possibility of inflammation.
- You could also take a 15-minute walk in the morning or at any time during the day.

You will significantly lower your stress. Make sure you get 7 full hours of sleep each night.

Take additional Magnesium, which relaxes the body. It is common nowadays to have a magnesium deficiency. Magnesium is considered the relaxation mineral.

There is a new study out by a research group at UC Berkeley. It has been published in a book called **Why We Sleep**.[6]

I have also learned that taking Magnolia Bark will relax the body before you go to sleep. You can buy it on Amazon.

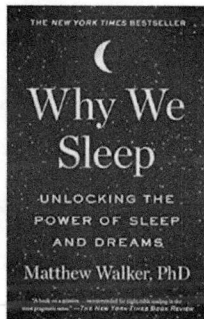

Dr. Walker considers it critical to get 7 hours of quality sleep each night for health. It cleans the plaque out of the brain that creates dementia. It allows your body to function with less stress during the day.

Your EVENING Routine

- Turn off all electronics 1/2 hour before bedtime
- Breathe to relax. I use the Dr. Andrew Weil 4-7-8 breathing exercise.
- Lower the temperature in your house for sleeping. We lower our home to 68.
- Keep a pen and pad by your bedside. If you can't sleep write down your busy thoughts and release them to the universe to be solved in your sleep
- If you can't fall asleep, do the mindful exercise of "washing" each of your chakras and ground yourself to the earth.

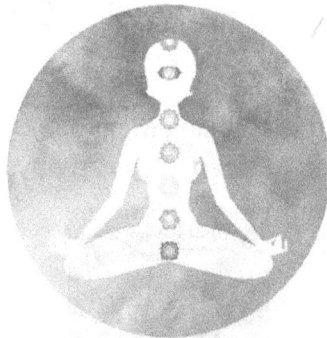

Start at the top of your head and bring light in through your 7th chakra, washing it in and out. Do this 3 times and then move the light down to your third eye, or your 6th chakra, and wash it in and out, now bring the light down to your 5th chakra, the throat and wash it front and back. Your throat chakra opens in both directions, now do down to your 4th chakra your heart and wash it in and out, now down to your 3rd chakra, your solar plexus and wash it in and out. Now bring the light to your 2nd chakra and wash it in and out and then down to your root chakra, now take the light straight down into the earth, lay roots as you go but keep the light going downwards until it reaches the core of the earth with is a very bright yellow light, enjoy the warmth and breathe for a count of 3, using the breathing in for 4, holding for 7 and whooshing it out for a count of 8. Now start bringing the light back up, and through all the roots you have laid in the earth until you reach the surface. Then bring the light up into your root chakra, your 2nd chakra, your solar plexus, your heart chakra, your throat chakra, your third eye, and now out your 7th chakra letting the light shower down your body. Now swirl the light around your body counter-clockwise and then clockwise, feeling the protection and the warmth of the light. Now relax. Usually, I am asleep long before I finish this exercise. I also use this exercise to protect myself.

Foster Weekly Alone time as part of your Stress care

- Spend Time Daily in Silence
- Mix your alone time with productivity, relaxation, and meditation or self-reflection.
- Go out into nature, where you'll have some of your deepest and most pure thoughts.
- The more time you spend with yourself and fill it with intentional productivity, self-care, and love, solitude will change from a generally lonely feeling into a positive time of growth in your life.
- Foster your "alone time." Once you go through the window of lonely to aloneness, you will savor your alone time. You will not be lonely again.
- Go find a beautiful tree and breathe with it. Take in its oxygen and give it your carbon dioxide.
- Hug the tree and get quiet. Ask it a question and listen for its answer. If you listen, you will hear it.

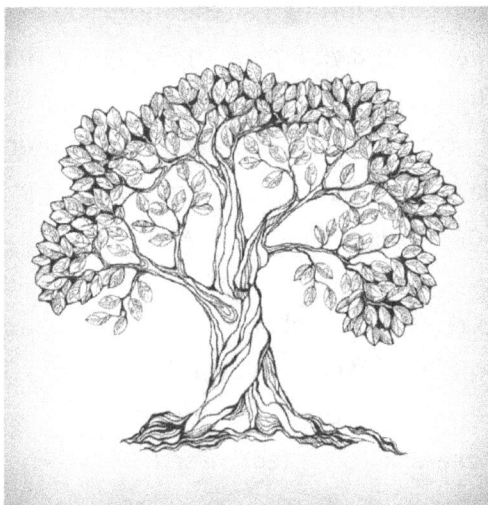

Using all these techniques on a regular basis will make you happier and more productive. Don't forget to laugh often and full. It may be the best stress-buster of all.

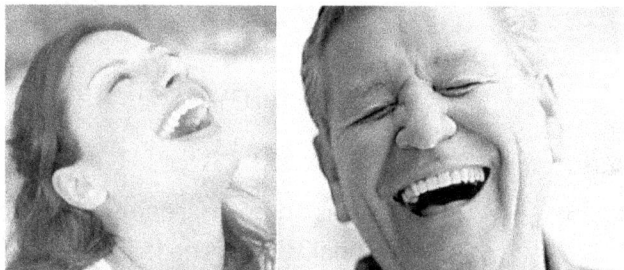

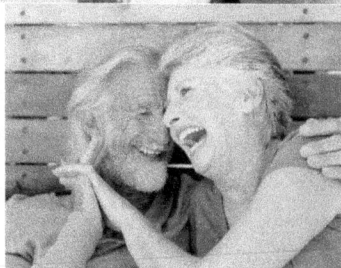

More about Cheryl

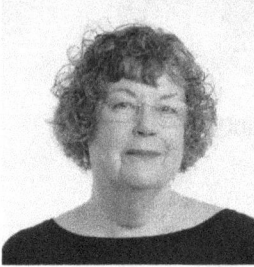

Cheryl Meyer aka Cheryl M Health Muse

Cheryl is an entrepreneur and Type A personality. For the last 20 years, she has owned a sterling silver jewelry company where she designed jewelry for major retailers. Previously, she was a VP/General Store Manager for a major department store where she managed and coached over 200 employees to be their best.

Cheryl is as Integrative Nutrition Health Coach, aka Cheryl M Health Muse. She is a self-published author and an anti-toxin advocate.

Why did she become a health muse? To put it simply, Cheryl got sick, very sick. She had terrible pain from autoimmune disease and wasn't finding answers. She spent five years researching focusing on toxins in her life and ways to lower chronic stress. Having returned to relative wellness, she wants to share what she has learned to help you.

What can this health muse do for you? Cheryl will inspire you to take charge of your life and reduce your pain. She will help you find the answers you need for wellness. She wants her journey back to health to inspire you in your journey. Cheryl has a mission. She wants to help you to discover how to live clean and eat clean in a toxic world.

Cheryl is a newlywed (at a ripe old age) and married for five years to her perfect match in the greater Pasadena, California area. Together she and John have also now purchased a home in The Village of Oak Creek, Sedona, AZ, which they now spend half their time. Being in Sedona helps Cheryl slow down and find balance. John is the editor of her books and the producer of her TV shows and podcasts.

Cheryl happily reports, now in my 70's "I FEEL GREAT AGAIN, and so can you! I feel better than I did in my 50's."

Cheryl is available for individual and group coaching as well as public speaking and workshops. You can contact her at cherylnhealthmuse@gmail.com and follow her on Facebook as Cherylmhealthmuse. Join her private Facebook group, Feeling Good, Living Low Toxin.

Want to be the first to know? Follow what she is doing next and stay informed with the latest and the greatest new information. Her newsletters and blogs are all about living the good life pain-free without toxins and without deprivation and her tricks and tips to live low toxin and feel great. It's easy to join her mailing list from any page on her website, which is also robust with great health information.

Watch her TV show on KGEM and KMAC community access TV in Monrovia, CA, Duarte, and Baldwin Park, CA. You can also watch the TV Episodes on her YouTube channel CherylMHealthMuse. You can find her books and shows on her new website heavenlytreepress.com, her publishing company website. She has her coaching and speaking website cherylmhealthmuse.com as well. Both offer valuable information to help you live your best, healthiest life.

Starting May 2020 watch for Cheryl's upcoming podcast, **It Feels Good to Feel Good, Futureproof your Health** and **Tell Me Your Story. The Health Muse is In** on RHG TV/Voice America. In the second part of her podcast, she will be interviewing others who have chronic illness and have also returned to wellness by making significant lifestyle changes. Cheryl wants to inspire you to do the same by listening to many success stories.

Her first book**, It Feels Good to Feel Good, Learn to Eliminate Toxins, Reduce Inflammation and Feel Great Again** has won 13 awards. It was revised and released as a second edition, Winter/Spring 2020. **H**er second book **is** a blueprint for living low toxin in everyday life. She also has a Victory and Gratitude Journal available on Amazon. This is Cheryl's third book**,** a pocketbook on Stress - 3-minute stress exercises to release stress before it becomes chronic to improve daily productivity. This book is designed to keep on your desk where you work so that it is handy to choose a 2-minute exercise whenever you need to release the steam off your stress. She is also planning a cookbook, **It Feels Good to Eat the Rainbow - recipes to cook with all the colors of fruits and vegetables for optimal health**. She plans to publish that in the Fall of 2020. Be on the lookout for her magazine in Sept 2020, where she will highlight guests from her podcast or who has made lifestyle changes to return to health. Cheryl is available for one on one coaching or for group coaching, either in her office in Monrovia, CA or by Zoom.

Call her today. 626 399 2304 or email her at cherylmhealthmuse@gmail.com.

Videos by Cheryl Meyer

Future Proof Your Health - TV Shows are made in cooperation with KGEM, Monrovia, CA. (2020)

Produced by John Gins.

Filmed by Chris Luiten, Operations Manager at KGEM-TV.

Special thank you to David Palomares, Executive Director at KGEM-TV, for all his support to make this a reality.

Future Proof Your Health Videos (2020)

Episode 1: The Benefits of Practicing Gratitude
Episode 2: The Importance of Releasing Stress
Episode 3: Conventional vs. GMO vs. Organic
Episode 4: You are What you Eat
Episode 5: Eat the Rainbow
Episode 6: Get to Know your Farmer's Market
Episode 7: 30 Ways to Save on Healthy Food
Episode 8: Turn Any Recipe Healthy
Episode 9: Eating Healthy Out in Restaurants
Episode 10: The Wonders of Trees

For more information https://heavenlytreepress.com

Cheryl is also available for corporate speaking.

Top subjects that she speaks on:

- It Feels Good to Feel Good - Future Proof Your Health - 12 things to start doing today.
- Food Quality Matters - Breaking the Confusion About Food. What SHOULD You Be Eating for Your Health and Your Family's Health?
- If Only I Had Wonder Woman's

Superpowers - Fighting Dr. Poison and the Duke of Deception (Where are the poisons and toxins in your life? What can you replace them with?)
- Lose Weight Without Dieting - Count Toxic Chemicals, Not Calories, and Learn the Keys to Unlock Weight Loss.
- Toxic Stress - Simple Exercises to Significantly Reduce it and improve productivity.

You can see her demo tape on YouTube.com. https://www.youtube.com/watch?v=56lGI9myYRM&t=11s

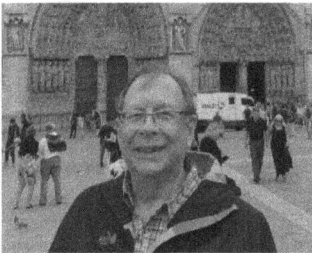

John Gins, Co-Author, and Editor

John is an officer of CherylMhealthMuse.com and Heavenly Tree Press. The mission of these companies is to help people be aware of the everyday toxins that we are all exposed to and what remedies can be taken to overcome exposure. John is the producer, editor, and technical support for the videos and books offered by Heavenly Tree Press. He provides Cheryl technical assistance for her online store.

His immediate interest is to help find ways to overcome the toxic lack of movement that has become prevalent in our society's sedentary lifestyle.

Before retiring in 2016, John worked in both applied statistics and computer technology for 43 years. In the Statistics arena, John wrote the prototype for CART in the '70s. This method for deriving decision trees from data is considered one of the earliest tools within the data mining community. Because of the computational demands of such automated statistical tools, John broadened his scope beyond statistics and consulting to computer systems and databases. John primarily consulted within the retail, financial, government, real estate, and internet industries. John is the primary author or significant contributor in over twenty publications.

John holds a BS in Mathematical Statistics from the University of Dayton and an MS in Mathematics from Wright State University in Dayton, Ohio.

John and Cheryl are ideal partners. They have been married now for five years.

What people have said about Cheryl's books

It Feels Good to Feel Good, Learn to Eliminate Toxins, Reduce Inflammation and Feel Great Again is now the recipient of 13 Book awards. Buy it today and see what all the buzz is about. https://cherylmhealthmuse.com/book/. You can also purchase it on Amazon. http://bit.ly/itfeelsgoodeliminatetoxins.

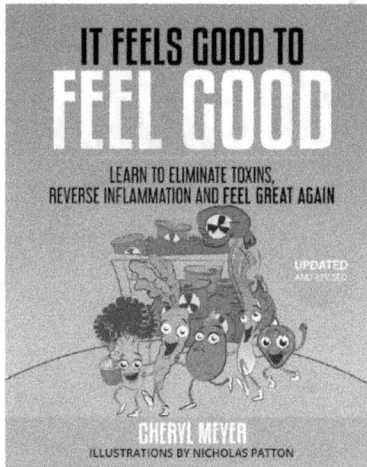

It comes with a workbook upon request. http://bit.ly/workbookitfeelsgood

---

"Amazing! Amazing! Amazing! I first want to say thank you and (big hugs). Your book may have saved my life. I'm 45 years old and have been struggling with unanswered symptoms for at least 5 years, and all conventional doctors want to do is wash me away with medication. You have saved some of the best years of my life with your information. Thank you so much." Lisa

---

"Your book and website have been very helpful in guiding my next steps while providing a beacon of hope for my fibromyalgia." With gratitude and peace, Rachel H

Hi Cheryl,
I first want to say thank you and (big hugs). Your book may have saved my life. I won your book btw and would love to praise it if there is a link (Goodreads).
I went to all of my conventional doctors, and not one would do any food testing. They all wanted to give me medication based on my symptoms. So, I turned to functional doctors, as you described in your book, and I found an amazing one about 45 minutes away. While I have to pay out of pocket for the visits, my insurance actually paid for the lab testing. All of my "normal" lab testing that a functional doctor would do came back well "normal," but the amount of information line by line, my functional doctor, gave me was amazing. Moving on to food sensitivity, I am blown away. I honestly don't know what I can eat. My card I take to a restaurant will probably be a small list of 3 things I can eat. Lol. From dairy to gluten to eggs to nuts, my panel is in the hot zone. No wonder every time I eat, I feel bad. Now because of that, both my functional and conventional doctor both

want me to see a GI doctor and have an endoscopy just to be sure we can see the whole picture, and that's coming next week.

After the results, my conventional doctors will sit down with me with the full case AND get this and with a nutritionist to map out a plan for three months starting to work with me. Based on my food panel, the nutritionist will be my best friend (I pray). Based on initial results, my conventional doctors suspect leaky gut and want a completely clean diet.

So, in summary, for now, you rock for writing your book! Maybe you've saved some of the best years of my life to come. I will keep in touch during and after these three months a D my journey ahead. Without your book, I would have never known about any of this. But I knew it had to be food just didn't understand any of it until now (well at least I'm starting).

Happy new year to you!!! And (hugs) (hugs) (hugs). Lisa

Reviewed in the United States on April 8, 2020
Format: Paperback

I loved how Cheryl invites us to make practical changes in our home environment gradually by replacing an item with a better alternative and not just throwing everything out at once. It is all a very doable strategy, and one she shares took her 5 years.

I loved learning about the effects of food and how literally we can use food to heal. Cheryl has a vast breadth of knowledge that she shares in a fun and

easy to understand way. She invites us to cook and eat real food from all the colors of the rainbow.
I have employed several of her suggestions about food and personal care products, and my awareness of the products I use in my home and environment has been raised. So grateful for the wisdom in this book. Enjoy. Janette Stuart

---

I have been dealing with Ulcerative Colitis for over 10 years, so I have tried a wide variety of different natural remedies and lifestyle alternatives. I struggle with reading traditional health books due to small fonts and getting overwhelmed with terminology.
Cheryl's book was highly informative but also engaging and fun to read due to her illustrations and digestible content. I quickly learned how to remove toxins from multiple areas of my life, and my Colitis symptoms improved drastically.
In addition to her book, Cheryl has gone out of her way to spend time on the phone with me to further educate me on helping my parents to have a better quality of life due to their ages and various conditions.
Cheryl is sincerely passionate about helping people to live a healthier lifestyle and not just "selling" her product/services.
Thank you!
Bryan Gallinger

"If you want to truly feel better, clean up! Just one tip from Cheryl's book will change your life. She has written the ultimate source for getting well through detoxification." Suzy Cohen, RPh Author of **Drug**

Muggers: Which Medications Are Robbing Your Body of Essential Nutrients and How to Restore Them.

"You have taken putting soap in the mouth for naughty words ..." to a New Level! LOL Who knew we were surrounded by so many toxins.
I've pretty much finished your book now working on giving sections to my family and friend that I think will especially appreciate certain chapters! YOU, my Dear, have found your calling, YOU make this rather "dull" subject a Very Good, interesting read, with fun personal touches along the way.
I LOVE your book; I hope people will embrace it. Why worry so much about health care if we keep killing ourselves with poison. We can all start with eliminating the toxins out of our lives. Val Peterson

---

This book takes you through step by step on how to eliminate toxins in your body, environment, and life. The author, Cheryl Meyer, understands that it takes time to make these changes and encourages the reader to make small changes to start.
Elimination of sugar is a vital course of action, but it is so difficult to do because there is sugar hidden in so many things. The book alerts you to how many added chemicals and unnecessary ingredients are in our "food" and demonstrates ways to eat more whole foods to improve overall health. I like that I can pick it up and review a relevant chapter at any time. Cosmetics were something I never thought of being a cause of toxins in our bodies! Eye-opening! Thank you, Cheryl! Gail Ross

Early reviews about **Feel Good, Living Low Toxin in Community and Everyday Life**

Once again Cheryl Meyer has captured a truly educational masterpiece every reader will benefit from, enjoy and gain valuable insight into the ever-challenging world we live. In her most recent book, **Feeling Good Living Low Toxin in Community and Everyday Life** Cheryl exposes the problem, provides practical solutions, executable action steps work for everyone suffering with unexplained inflammatory conditions and illnesses MUST read. As a Naturopath with over 30k clinical hours of hands on experience helping sick people get well, Cheryl's book is now on my Must-read list for all patients in my practice. Thank you for your amazing contribution!
Dan Young, BCN, CNC
AANWP/ANMCB Nationally Board-Certified Naturopath
Clinician/Speaker/Author

ENDNOTES

[1] Meyer, Cheryl, **It Feels Good to Feel Good, Learn to Eliminate Toxins, Reduce Inflammation and Feel Great Again,** Heavenly Tree Press 2020, You can also purchase it on Amazon. http://bit.ly/itfeelsgoodeliminatetoxins

[2] https://www.news-medical.net/life-sciences/Telomere-What-are- Telomeres.aspx

[3] https://www.etsy.com/listing/206233427/salute-the-sun-blank-yoga- pose-greeting?ref=internal_similar_listing_bot-12&frs=1

[4] https://juliacameronlive.com/basic-tools/morning-pages/

[5] https://www.bellybuttonhealing.com/

[6] https://www.amazon.com/Why-We-Sleep-Unlocking-Dreams/dp/1501144316/ref=sr_1_3?keywords=why+we+sleep&qid=1556394430&s=gateway&sr=8-3